The 55 Best

Plant-Based Recipes

Everything you Need to Know to Prepare Your Favorite

The Green Solution

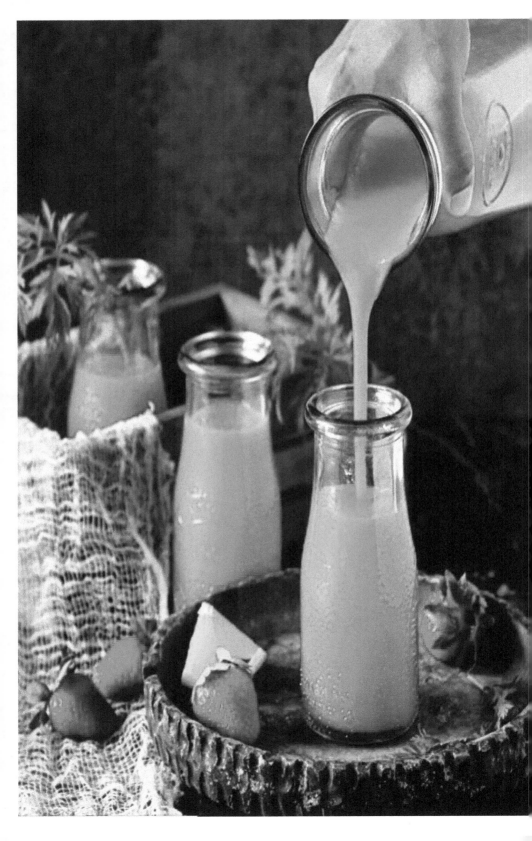

Table of Contents

INTRODUCTION

A plant-based diet is a diet consisting mostly or entirely of plant-based foods with no animal products or artificial ingredients. While a plant-based diet avoids or has limited animal products, it is not necessarily vegan. This includes not only fruits and vegetables, but also nuts, seeds, oils, whole grains, legumes, and beans. It doesn't mean that you are vegetarian or vegan and never eat meat, eggs, or dairy.

Vegetarian diets have also been shown to support health, including a lower risk of developing coronary heart disease, high blood pressure, diabetes, and increased longevity.

Plant-based diets offer all the necessary carbohydrates, vitamins, protein, fats, and minerals for optimal health, and are often higher in fiber and phytonutrients. However, some vegans may need to add a supplement to ensure they receive all the nutrients required.

Who says that plant-based diets are limited or boring? There are lots of delicious recipes that you can use to make mouthwatering, healthy, plant-based dishes that will satisfy your cravings. If you're eating these plant-based foods regularly, you can maintain a healthy weight without obsessing about calories and avoid diseases that result from bad dietary habits.

Benefits of a Plant-Based Diet

Eating a plant-based diet improves the health of your gut so you are better able to absorb the nutrients from food that support your immune system and reduce inflammation. Fiber can lower cholesterol and stabilize blood sugar, and it's great for good bowel management.

- **A Plant-Based Diet May Lower Your Blood Pressure**
  High blood pressure, or hypertension, can increase the risk for health issues, including heart disease, stroke, and type 2 diabetes and reduce blood pressure and other risky conditions.

- **A Plant-Based Diet May Keep Your Heart Healthy**
  Saturated fat in meat can contribute to heart issues when eaten in excess, so plant-based foods can help keep your heart healthy.

- **A Plant-Based Diet May Help Prevent Type 2 Diabetes**
  Animal foods can increase cholesterol levels, so eating a plant-based diet filled with high-quality plant foods can reduce the risk of developing type 2 diabetes by 34 percent.

- **Eating a Plant-Based Diet Could Help You Lose Weight**
  Cutting back on meat can help you to maintain a healthy weight because a plant-based diet is naturally satisfying and rich in fiber.

- **Following a Plant-Based Diet Long Term May Help You Live Longer**

  If you stick with healthy plant-based foods your whole body will be leaner and healthier, allowing you to stay healthy and vital as you age.

- **A Plant-Based Diet May Decrease Your Risk of Cancer**

  Vegetarians have an 18 percent lower risk of cancer compared to non-vegetarians. This is because a plant-based diet is rich of fibers and healthy nutrients.

- **A Plant-Based Diet May Improve Your Cholesterol**

  High cholesterol can lead to fatty deposits in the blood, which can restrict blood flow and potentially lead to heart attack, stroke, heart disease, and many other problems. A plant-based diet can help in maintaining healthy cholesterol levels.

- **Ramping Up Your Plant Intake May Keep Your Brain Strong**

  Increased consumption of fruits and vegetables is associated with a 20 percent reduction in the risk of cognitive impairment and dementia. So plant foods can help protect your brain from multiple issues.

What to Eat in Plant-Based Diets

Fruits: Berries, citrus fruits, pears, peaches, pineapple, bananas, etc.

Vegetables: Kale, spinach, tomatoes, broccoli, cauliflower, carrots, asparagus, peppers, etc.

Starchy vegetables: Potatoes, sweet potatoes, butternut squash, etc.

Whole grains: Brown rice, rolled oats, farro, quinoa, brown rice pasta, barley, etc.

Healthy fats: Avocados, olive oil, coconut oil, unsweetened coconut, etc.

Legumes: Peas, chickpeas, lentils, peanuts, black beans, etc.

Seeds, nuts, and nut butters: Almonds, cashews, macadamia nuts, pumpkin seeds, sunflower seeds, natural peanut butter, tahini, etc.

Unsweetened plant-based milks: Coconut milk, almond milk, cashew milk, etc.

Spices, herbs, and seasonings: Basil, rosemary, turmeric, curry, black pepper, salt, etc.

Condiments: Salsa, mustard, nutritional yeast, soy sauce, vinegar, lemon juice, etc.

Plant-based protein: Tofu, tempeh, plant-based protein sources or powders with no added sugar or artificial ingredients.

Beverages: Coffee, tea, sparkling water, etc.

What Not to Eat in Plant-Based Diets

Fast food: French fries, cheeseburgers, hot dogs, chicken nuggets, etc.

Added sugars and sweets: Table sugar, soda, juice, pastries, cookies, candy, sweet tea, sugary cereals, etc.

Refined grains: White rice, white pasta, white bread, bagels, etc.

Packaged and convenience foods: Chips, crackers, cereal bars, frozen dinners, etc.

Processed vegan-friendly foods: Plant-based meats like; Tofurkey, faux cheeses, vegan butters, etc.

Artificial sweeteners: Equal, Splenda, Sweet'N Low, etc.

Processed animal products: Bacon, lunch meats, sausage, beef jerky, etc.

Day 1:

Breakfast (304 calories)

- 1 serving Berry-Kefir Smoothie

A.M. Snack (95 calories)

- 1 medium apple

Lunch (374 calories)

- 1 serving Green Salad with Pita Bread & Hummus

P.M. Snack (206 calories)

- 1/4 cups dry-roasted unsalted almonds

Dinner (509 calories)

- 1 serving Beefless Vegan Tacos
- 2 cups mixed greens
- 1 serving Citrus Vinaigrette

Day 2:

Breakfast (258 calories)

- 1 serving Cinnamon Roll Overnight Oats
- 1 medium orange

A.M. Snack (341 calories)

- 1 cup low-fat plain Greek yogurt
- 1 medium peach
- 3 tbsps slivered almonds

Lunch (332 calories)

- 1 serving Thai-Style Chopped Salad with Sriracha Tofu

P.M. Snack (131 calories)

- 1 large pear

Dinner (458 calories)

- 1 serving Mexican Quinoa Salad

Day 3:

Breakfast (258 calories)

- 1 serving Cinnamon Roll Overnight Oats
- 1 medium orange

A.M. Snack (95 calories)

- 1 medium apple

Lunch (463 calories)

- 1 serving Thai-Style Chopped Salad with Sriracha Tofu
- 1 large pear

P.M. Snack (274 calories)

- 1/3 cups dried walnut halves
- 1 medium peach

Dinner (419 calories)

- 1 serving Eggs in Tomato Sauce with Chickpeas & Spinach
- 1 1-oz. slice whole-wheat baguette

SMOOTHIES & BREAKFAST

Homemade Hearty Smoothie

Servings: 6

Preparation Time: 5 minutes

Ingredients:

- ½ tsp ground cinnamon
- 1 cup coconut milk
- 1 tbsp fresh ginger
- 1 cup water
- 2 bananas
- 4 cherries, pitted
- 1/2 tsp cardamom
- 2 cups broccoli sprouts
- 2 tbsps hemp hearts

Procedure:

1. First, in a food processor, place banana, coconut milk, water, broccoli, cherries, hemp hearts, cinnamon, cardamom, and ginger.
2. Then blitz until smooth.
3. After that, divide between glasses and serve.

Tasty Carrot-Strawberry Smoothie

Servings: 4

Preparation Time: 5 minutes

Ingredients:

- 4 tbsps maple syrup
- 4 cups sweetened almond milk
- 2 cups strawberries
- 2 apples chopped
- 2 peeled and diced carrots

Procedure:

1. First, place in a food processor all the ingredients.
2. Now blitz until smooth.
3. Finally, pour in glasses and serve.

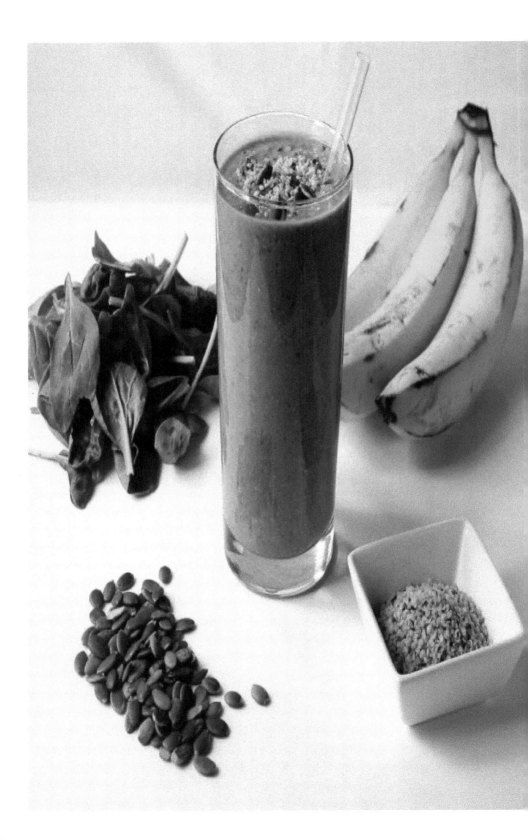

Healthy chia-peach smoothie

Servings: 4

Preparation Time: 5 minutes

Ingredients:

- 2 bananas, sliced
- 2 cups almond milk
- 2 cucumbers chopped
- 2 peaches chopped
- 2 scoops plant-based protein powder
- 2 tbsps Chia seeds

Procedure:

1. First, put the bananas, peaches, almond milk, protein powder, chia seeds, and cucumbers in a food processor.
2. Now blend it until smooth.
3. Lastly, serve immediately in glasses.

Delicious Morning Green Smoothie

Servings: 4

Preparation Time: 5 minutes

Ingredients:

- 4 apples peeled and cored
- 2 cups unsweetened coconut yogurt
- 4 cups curly endive
- 4 tbsps Lime juice
- 4 tbsps Chia seeds
- 2 avocados
- 4 cups soy milk
- 2 cups chopped cucumber
- 1 inch piece peeled fresh ginger

Procedure:

1. First, put in a food processor the avocados, cucumber, curly endive, apple, lime juice, soy milk, ginger, chia seeds, and coconut yogurt.
2. Then blend until smooth
3. Lastly, serve.

Fry bread with Peanut Butter and Jam

Servings: 6

Preparation Time: 20 minutes

Per serving: Calories: 293; Fat: 7.8g; Carbs: 50.3g; Protein: 5.5g

Ingredients:

- 1 cup warm water
- 1 teaspoon baking powder
- 1 teaspoon coconut sugar
- 6 tablespoons raspberry jam
- 2 cups all-purpose flour
- 1 teaspoon sea salt
- 6 teaspoons peanut butter
- 6 teaspoons olive oil

Procedure:

1. First, thoroughly combine the flour, baking powder, salt, and sugar.
2. Now gradually add in the water until the dough comes together.
3. Then divide the dough into three balls; flatten each ball to create circles.
4. Heat 1 teaspoon of olive oil in a frying pan over a moderate flame.
5. After that, fry the first bread for about 9 minutes or until golden brown.

6. Then repeat with the remaining oil and dough.
7. Finally, serve the fry bread with peanut butter and raspberry jam. Enjoy!

Tasty Ciabatta Bread Pudding with Sultanas

Servings: 8

Preparation Time: 2 hours 10 minutes

Per serving: Calories: 458; Fat: 10.4g; Carbs: 81.3g; Protein: 11.4g

Ingredients:

- 1 cup sultana raisins
- 4 cups coconut unsweetened milk
- ½ teaspoon ground cloves
- ½ teaspoon himalayan salt
- 1 1/2 pounds stale ciatta bread, cubed
- 1 cup agave syrup
- 1 teaspoon ground cardamom
- 1 teaspoon ground cinnamon
- 1 teaspoon vanilla essence
- 2 tablespoons coconut oil

Procedure:

1. First, in a mixing bowl, combine the coconut milk, agave syrup, coconut oil, vanilla, cardamom, ground cloves, cinnamon, and Himalayan salt.
2. Now add the bread cubes to the custard mixture and stir to combine well.
3. Then fold in the sultana raisins and allow it to rest for about 1 hour on a counter.

4. Then, spoon the mixture into a lightly oiled casserole dish.
5. After that, bake in the preheated oven at 350 degrees F for about 1 hour or until the top is golden brown.
6. Lastly, place the bread pudding on a wire rack for 10 minutes before slicing and serving. Bon app tit!

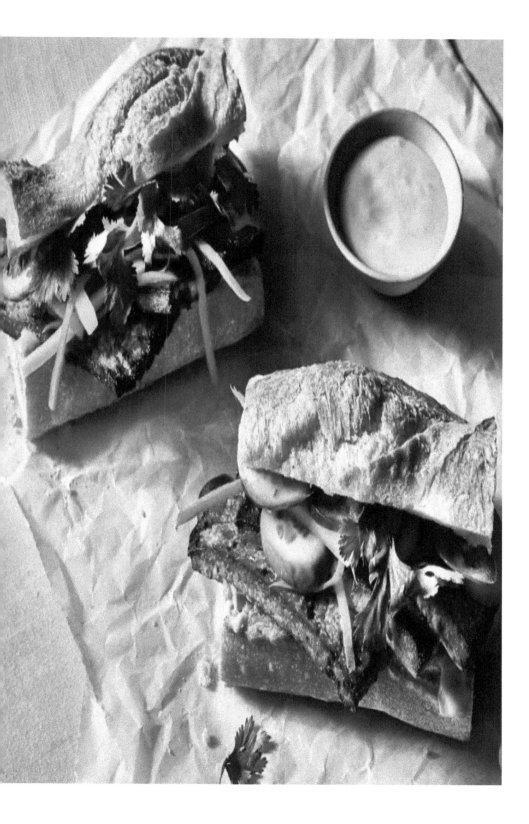

Homemade Vegan Banh Mi

Servings: 8

Preparation Time: 35 minutes

Per serving: Calories: 372; Fat: 21.9g; Carbs: 29.5g;
Protein: 17.6g

Ingredients:

- 8 lime wedges
- 8 tablespoons fresh cilantro chopped
- 4 standard french baguettes, cut into four pieces
- Koshar salt and ground black pepper to taste
- ½ cup fresh parsley chopped
- 4 cloves of garlic minced
- 3 tablespoons soya sauce
- ½ cup vegan mayonnaise
- 24 ounces firm tofu cut into sticks
- 4 tablespoons olive oil
- 2 white onions thinly sliced
- 1 cup white radish cut into 1/6 -inch -thick matchsticks
- 4 carrots cut into 1/6 -inch -thick matchsticks
- ½ cup white sugar
- ½ cup water
- 1 cup rice vinegar

Procedure:

1. First, bring the rice vinegar, water, and sugar to a boil and stir until the sugar has dissolved for about 1 minute.
2. Now allow it to cool. Pour the cooled vinegar mixture over the carrot, daikon radish, and onion; allow the vegetables to marinate for at least 30 minutes.
3. While the vegetables are marinating, heat the olive oil in a frying pan over medium-high heat.
4. Once hot, add the tofu and sauté for 8 minutes, occasionally stirring to promote even cooking.
5. Then, mix the mayo, soy sauce, garlic, parsley, salt, and ground black pepper in a small bowl. Slice each piece of the baguette in half the long way
6. Then, toast the baguette halves under the preheated broiler for about 3 minutes.
7. To assemble the banh mi sandwiches, spread each half of the toasted baguette with the mayonnaise mixture; fill the cavity of the bottom half of the bread with the fried tofu sticks, marinated vegetables and cilantro leaves.
8. Lastly, squeeze the lime wedges over the filling and top with the other half of the baguette.

Homemade Chocolate Peppermint Mousse

Servings: 4

Preparation Time: 10minutes, 30minutes refrigeration

Per Serving: Calories: 70, Total Fat7.4: g, Saturated Fat: 4.6g, Total Carbs: 1g, Dietary Fiber: 0g, Sugar: 0 g, Protein: 0g, Sodium: 8 mg

Ingredients:

- 2/3 cup coconut cream
- 8 oz. dairy-free cashew cream softened
- 1 tsp vanilla extract
- 1/2 cup swerve sugar, divided
- 6 tbsps unsweetened cocoa powder
- 1/2 cup of warm water
- 2/4 tsp peppermint extract

Procedure:

1. Put 2 tablespoons of swerve sugar, the cashew cream, and cocoa powder in a blender.
2. Now add the peppermint extract, warm water, and process until smooth.
3. Take a large bowl; whip the vanilla extract, coconut cream, and the remaining swerve sugar using a whisk.
4. Then fetch out 5 to 6 tablespoons for garnishing.

5. Next, fold in the cocoa mixture until thoroughly combined.
6. Now spoon the mousse into serving cups and chill in the fridge for 30 minutes.
7. Lastly, garnish with the reserved whipped cream and serve immediately.

Healthy Morning Nutty Oatmeal Muffins

Serving: 18

Preparation Time: 30 minute

Per serving: Calories: 192; Fat: 6g; Carbs: 30.5g; Protein: 5.6g

Ingredients:
- 1 cup shredded coconut, unsweetened
- 1 1/2 teaspoons baking powder
- 1/2 teaspoon salt
- 1/2 cup pecans, chopped
- 1/2 teaspoon vanilla extract
- 3 cups rolled oats
- 1/2 teaspoon coconut extract
- 1 teaspoon cardamom
- 1/2 teaspoon grated nutmeg
- 1 1/2 cups coconut milk
- 2/3 cup canned pumpkin
- 1/2 cup agave syrup
- 1/2 cup golden raisins

Procedure:

1. Begin by preheating your oven to 360 degrees F.
2. Now spritz a muffin tin with nonstick cooking oil.
3. Then in a mixing bowl, thoroughly combine all the ingredients, except for the raisins and pecans.

4. After that, fold in the raisins and pecans and scrape the batter into the prepared muffin tin.
5. Finally, bake your muffins for about 25 minutes or until the top is set. Bon appétit!

Amazing Raspberry and Chia Smoothie Bowl

Servings: 4

Preparation Time: 10 minutes

Per Serving: Calories: 442; Fat: 10.9g; Carbs: 85g; Protein: 9.6g

Ingredients:

- 4 tablespoons chia seeds
- 2 tablespoons pepitas
- 2 tablespoons coconut flakes
- 4 dates, pitted
- 3 cups raspberries, fresh or frozen
- 4 small sized bananas peeled
- 2 cups coconut milk

Procedure:

1. First, in your blender or food processor, mix the coconut milk with the bananas, raspberries, and dates.
2. Now process until creamy and smooth.
3. Then divide the smoothie between two bowls.
4. Finally, top each smoothie bowl with the coconut flakes, pepitas, and chia seeds. Bon appétit!

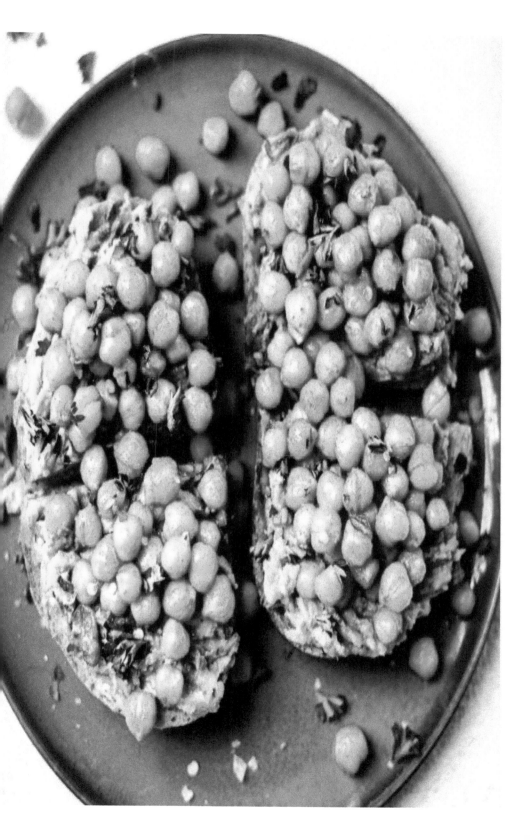

Healthy and Tasty Chickpeas Spread Sourdough Toast

Servings: 8

Preparation Time: 15-30 minutes

Per Serving: Carbs: 33. 7g Protein: 8. 45g Fats: 2. 5g Calories: 187Kcal

Ingredients:

- 4 slices toasted sourdough
- Salt as per taste
- 1 cup vegan yogurt
- 2 cups pumpkin
- 2 cups rinsed and drained chickpeas

Procedure:

1. First, in a bowl, add chickpeas and pumpkin puree and mash using a potato masher.
2. Then add in salt and yogurt and mix.
3. Now spread it on a toast and serve.

Healthy Keto Brownies

Servings: 4

Preparation Time: 10minutes

Per Serving:

Calories: 321, Total Fat: 40.3g, Saturated Fat: 18 g, Total Carbs: 19 g, Dietary Fiber: 5g, Sugar: 4 g, Protein: 2 g, Sodium: 265 mg

Ingredients:

- 4 oz. dairy-free dark chocolate
- 1/2 cup unsweetened cocoa powder
- 4 tbsps flax seed powder + 6 tbsp water
- 1 teaspoon vanilla extract optional
- 1 cup almond flour
- 1 tsp baking powder
- 1 cup erythritol
- 20 tablespoons butter 1 cup + 4 tbsps

Procedure:

1. Preheat the oven to 375 F and line a baking sheet with parchment paper. Set aside.
2. Now mix the flaxseed powder with water in a bowl and allow thickening for 5 minutes.
3. Take a separate bowl; mix the cocoa powder, almond flour, baking powder, and erythritol until no lumps from the erythritol remain.

4. Then in another bowl, now add the butter and dark chocolate and melt both in the microwave for 30 seconds to 1 minute.
5. Now whisk the flax egg and vanilla into the chocolate mixture, and then pour the mixture into the dry ingredients. Combine evenly.
6. Pour the batter onto the paper-lined baking sheet and bake in the oven for 20 minutes or until a toothpick inserted into the cake comes out clean.
7. After that, remove from the oven to cool completely and refrigerate for 30 minutes to 2 hours.
8. When ready, slice into squares, and serve.

SOUPS & STEWS

Delicious Pumpkin & Garbanzo Chili with Kale

Servings: 12

Preparation Time: 60 minutes

Ingredients:

- 1 tsp salt
- 6 cups kale, chopped
- 1 tsp garlic powder
- 2 tsps onion powder
- 2 tbsps chili powder
- 12 cups water
- 4 cups chopped pumpkin
- 2(56-oz) can crushed tomatoes
- 1 1/2 cups dried garbanzo beans, soaked

Procedure:

1. First, in a saucepan over medium heat, add garbanzo, tomatoes, pumpkin, 2 cups water, salt, chili, onion, and garlic powders.
2. Now bring to a boil.
3. Reduce the heat and simmer for 50 minutes.
4. Then stir in kale and cook for 5 minutes until the kale wilts.
5. Finally, serve.

Special Spanish Gazpacho

Servings: 8

Preparation Time: 15 minutes

Ingredients:

- 4 tbsps chopped dill
- 2 cups tomato juice
- 2 (29-oz)can crushed tomatoes
- 4 lbs. ripe plum tomatoes chopped
- 4 tsps lemon juice
- 4 cucumbers
- Salt and black pepper to taste
- 4 garlic cloves crushed
- 6 tbsps olive oil

Procedure:

1. First, in a food processor, put the garlic, olive oil, and salt and pulse until paste-like consistency forms.
2. Now add in 1 cucumber and lemon juice.
3. After that, blitz until smooth.
4. Put in tomatoes, tomato juice, salt, and pepper.
5. Then blend until smooth.
6. In the end, transfer to a bowl, close the lid, and let chill in the fridge before serving.

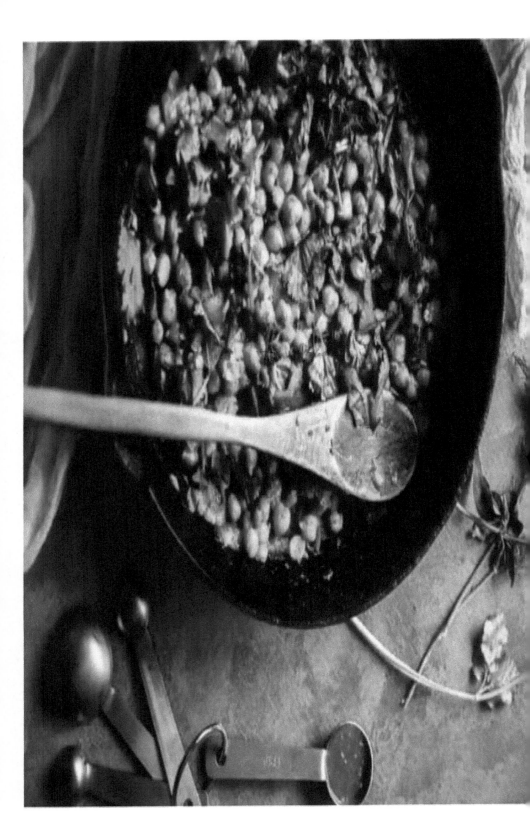

Special Chickpeas with Harissa

Servings: 4

Preparation Time: 15-30 minutes

Per Serving: Carbs: 55. 6 g Protein: 17. 8g Fats: 11. 8g
Calories: 398Kcal

Ingredients:

- 4 tsps Harissa
- 4 tbsps Lemon juice
- Salt as per your taste
- 2 cups diced tomatoes
- 2 cups diced cucumbers
- 2 small diced onions
- 2 cups can chickpeas
- 2 tbsps olive oil
- 4 tbsps chopped flat-leaf parsley

Procedure:

1. First, add lemon juice, harissa, and olive oil in a bowl and whisk.
2. Then take a serving bowl and add onion, cucumber, chickpeas, salt, and the sauce you made.
3. At last, add parsley from the top and serve.

Homemade Green Bean & Zucchini Veloute

Servings: 12

Preparation Time: 30 minutes

Ingredients:

- 6 medium zucchinis sliced
- 2 onions chopped
- 2 garlic cloves minced
- 8 cups vegetable broth
- 4 cups green beans
- 6 tbsps olive oil
- 4 tbsps minced jarred pimiento
- 1 tsp dried marjoram
- 1 cup plain almond milk

Procedure:

1. First, heat oil in a pot and sauté onion and garlic for 5 minutes.
2. Then add in green beans and broth.
3. Now cook for 10 minutes.
4. After that, stir in zucchini and cook for 10 minutes.
5. Hen transfer to a food processor and pulse until smooth.
6. Now return to the pot and mix in almond milk; cook until hot.
7. Finally, serve topped with pimiento.

Delicious Mushroom, Chickpea & Eggplant Stew

Servings: 8

Preparation Time: 30 minutes

Ingredients:

- 2 tbsps Soy sauce
- 2 tbsps minced parsley
- 1 tsp Dried oregano
- 1 tsp dried basil
- Salt and black pepper to taste
- 1 cup vegetable broth
- 4 tbsps olive oil
- 2 onions chopped
- 2 eggplants chopped
- 4 medium carrots sliced
- 2 red tomatoes chopped
- 2 cups mushrooms sliced
- 4 garlic cloves minced
- 2(31-oz) chickpeas can drained
- 2(56-oz) diced can tomatoes

Procedure:

1. First, heat the oil in a pot over medium heat.
2. Place in onion, garlic, eggplant, and carrots and sauté for 5 minutes.

3. Now lower the heat and stir in potato, mushrooms, chickpeas, tomatoes, oregano, basil, soy sauce, salt, pepper, and broth.
4. Then simmer for 15 minutes.
5. Lastly, serve sprinkled with parsley.

Delicious Grandma's Creamy Soup

Servings: 8

Preparation Time: 40 minutes

Per Serving: Calories: 400; Fat: 9.3g; Carbs: 72.5g; Protein: 9.3g

Ingredients:

- 2 cups coconut milk
- 6 cups vegetable broth
- 1 teaspoon mustard powder
- 1 teaspoon fennel seeds
- Koshar salt and cayenne pepper to taste
- 1 teaspoon ground cumin
- 4 garlic cloves
- 8 large potatoes, peeled and sliced
- 8 large carrots, trimmed and sliced
- 2 shallot chopped
- 4 tablespoons olive oil

Procedure:

1. Take a heavy-bottomed pot, heat the olive oil over medium-high heat.
2. Once hot, sauté the shallot, carrots, and potatoes for about 5 minutes, stirring periodically.
3. Now add in the garlic and continue to sauté for 1 minute or until fragrant.

4. Then, stir in the ground cumin, mustard powder, fennel seeds, salt, cayenne pepper, and vegetable broth; bring to a rapid boil.
5. After that, immediately reduce the heat to a simmer and let it cook for about 30 minutes.
6. Puree the soup using an immersion blender until creamy and uniform.
7. Then return the pureed soup to the pot.
8. Now fold in the coconut milk and continue to simmer until heated through or about 5 minutes longer.
9. Lastly, ladle into four bowls and serve hot.

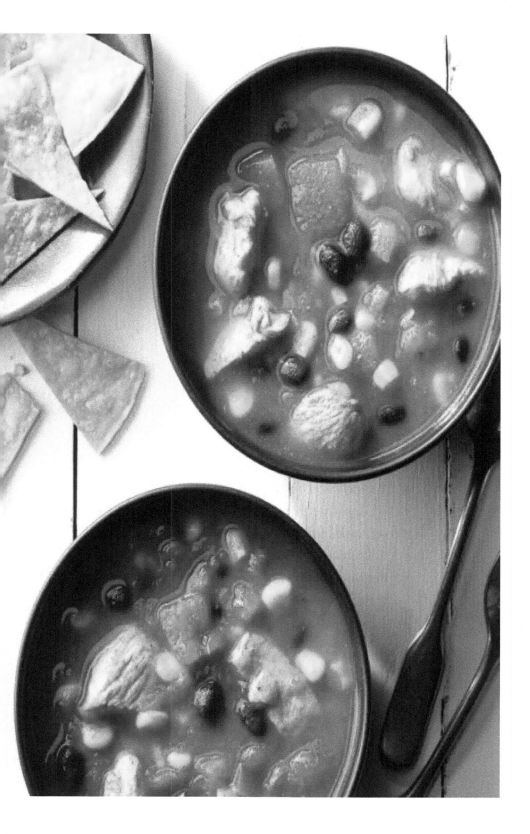

Mexican style Delicious chili soup

Servings: 8

Preparation Time: 1 hour and 15 minutes

Per serving: Calories: 498; Fat: 10.4g; Carbs: 74.9g; Protein: 28.3g

Ingredients:

- 2 bay laurel
- 4 tablespoons olive oil
- 2 medium-sized leek, chopped
- 1 teaspoon mustard seeds
- 4 red bell peppers, chopped
- 1 teaspoon cumin seeds
- 2 chipotle chili peppers, chopped
- 4 cloves of garlic, chopped
- 8 cups vegetable broth
- 4 cups dry red beans, soaked overnight and drained
- 4 ounces tortilla chips
- 1 teaspoon fennel seeds
- Kosher salt and ground black pepper, to taste
- 1 cup salsa
- 6 heaping tablespoons fresh cilantro, chopped

Procedure:

1. Start with placing the soaked beans in a soup pot; cover with a fresh change of the water and bring to

a boil over medium-high heat. Let it boil for about 10 minutes.

2. Next, turn the heat to a simmer and continue to cook for 45 minutes; reserve.
3. In the same pot, heat the olive over medium-high heat.
4. Now, sauté the leek and peppers for approximately 3 minutes or until the vegetables have softened.
5. Add in the chipotle chili pepper and garlic and continue to sauté for 1 minute or until aromatic.
6. Then, add in the vegetable broth, bay laurel, fennel seeds, mustard seeds, cumin seeds, salt, and black pepper and bring to a boil.
7. Immediately reduce the heat to a simmer and let it cook for 10 minutes.
8. Now fold in the reserved beans and continue to simmer for about 10 minutes longer until everything is thoroughly heated.
9. Lastly, ladle into individual bowls and serve with salsa, cilantro, and tortilla chips.

Homemade Green Lentil Stew with Brown Rice

Servings: 8

Preparation Time: 15-30 minutes

Per Serving: Calories 1305 kcal Fats 130. 9g Carbs 25. 1g Protein 24. 3g

Ingredients:

For the stew:

- 2 lbs. tempeh, cut into cubes
- 4 celery stalks, chopped
- 2 tsps chili powder
- 4 carrots diced
- 2 tsps onion powder
- 2 tsps cumin powder
- 2 tsps garlic powder
- 4 tbsps olive oil
- 2 limes, juiced
- 2 yellow onions, chopped
- Salt and black pepper to taste
- 8 garlic cloves, minced
- 4 cups vegetable broth
- 2 tsps oregano
- 2 cups green lentils, rinsed
- 1/2 cup chopped tomatoes

For the brown rice:

- Salt to taste
- 2 cups of brown rice
- 2 cups of water

Procedure:

1. First, heat the olive oil in a large pot, season the tempeh with salt, black pepper, and cook in the oil until brown, 10 minutes.
2. Now stir in the chili powder, onion powder, cumin powder, garlic powder, and cook until fragrant, 1 minute.
3. After that, mix in the onion, celery, carrots, garlic, and cook until softened.
4. Pour in the vegetable broth, oregano, green lentils, tomatoes, and green chilies.
5. Now cover the pot and cook until the tomatoes soften and the stew reduces by half, 10 to 15 minutes.
6. Open the lid, adjust the taste with salt, black pepper, and mix in the lime juice.
7. Then dish the stew and serve warm with the brown rice.
8. Meanwhile, as the stew cooks, add the brown rice, water, and salt to a medium pot.
9. Finally, cook over medium heat until the rice is tender and the water is absorbed for about 15 to 25 minutes.

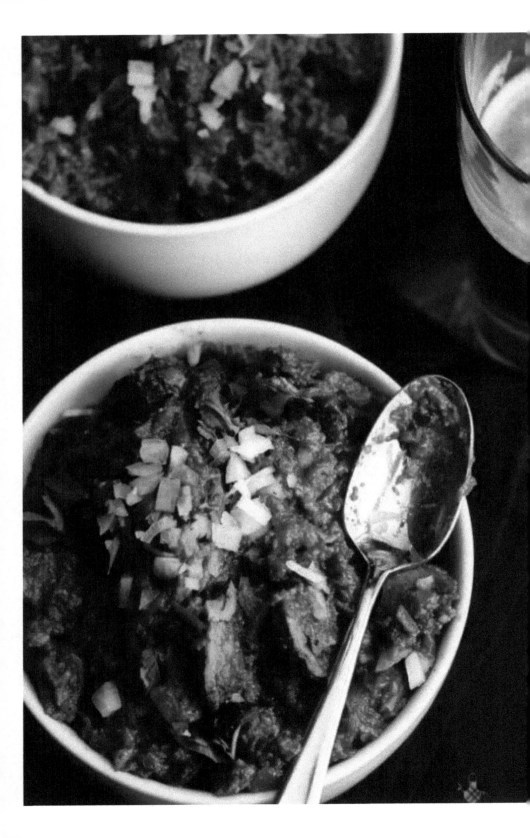

Special Chili Seitan Stew with Brown Rice

Servings: 8

Preparation Time: 15-30 minutes

Per Serving: Calories 1290 Fats 131. 8g Carbs 15. 2g Protein 24. 4g

Ingredients:

For the stew:

- Salt and black pepper to taste
- 2 tsps chili powder
- 2 tsps of onion powder
- 2 tsps of oregano
- 2 tsps cumin powder
- 2 tsps garlic powder
- 2 yellow onions, chopped
- 6 green chilies, deseeded and chopped
- 4 celeries stalks, chopped
- 4 tbsps olive oil
- 4 carrots diced
- 8 cloves garlic
- 2 lbs seitan, cut into cubes
- 2 cups vegetable broth
- 2 cups of water
- 2 cups chopped tomatoes

For the brown rice:

- Salt to taste
- 2 cups of brown rice
- 2 cups of water
- 2 limes, juiced

Procedure:

1. Firstly, heat the olive oil in a large pot, season the seitan with salt, black pepper, and cook in the oil until brown, 10 minutes.
2. Now stir in the chili powder, onion powder, cumin powder, garlic powder, and cook until fragrant, 1 minute.
3. After that, mix in the onion, celery, carrots, garlic, and cook until softened.
4. Pour in the vegetable broth, water, oregano, tomatoes, and green chilies.
5. Then cover the pot and cook until the tomatoes soften and the stew reduces by half, 10 to 15 minutes.
6. Now open the lid, adjust the taste with salt, black pepper, and mix in the lime juice.
7. Then dish the stew and serve warm with the brown rice.
8. Meanwhile, as the stew cooks, add the brown rice, water, and salt to a medium pot.
9. Finally, cook over medium heat until the rice is tender and the water absorbs 15 to 20 minutes.

Homemade Fruits Stew

Servings: 8

Preparation Time: 10 minutes

Per Serving: Calories 178, Fat 4.4, Fiber 2, Carbs 3, and Protein 5

Ingredients:

- 2 tablespoons lemon juice
- 4 tablespoons stevia
- 2 cups plums, stoned and halved
- 2 avocados, peeled, pitted, and sliced
- 4 teaspoons vanilla extract
- 4 cups of water

Procedure:

1. Take a pan, combine the avocado with the plums, water, and the other ingredients, bring to a simmer, and cook over medium heat for 10 minutes.
2. Now divide the mix into bowls and serve cold.

Homemade Vegan Tofu and Little Potato Stew

Servings: 10

Preparation Time: 10 minutes

Per Serving: Calories 152, Total Fat 7g, Saturated Fat 2g, Total Carbs 17g, Net Carbs 14g, Protein 6g, Sugar: 3g, Fiber: 3g, Sodium: 880mg, Potassium: 975mg, Phosphorus: 436mg

Ingredients:

- 2 block (700g) extra-firm tofu, cubed
- 6 tablespoons tomato paste
- 4 cloves of garlic
- 3 cups carrots
- 3 cups chopped celery
- 4 tablespoons cornstarch + 3 tablespoons water
- 3 pounds baby potatoes, scrubbed
- 2 cups frozen peas
- 4 tablespoons olive oil
- 4 tablespoons soy sauce
- 1 cup chopped yellow onion
- 2 cups of water
- salt and pepper to taste
- 12 cups vegetable broth

Procedure:

1. Start with pressing the Sauté button on the Instant Pot and heat the oil.
2. Now sear the tofu on all sides until lightly golden.
3. Stir in the onion and garlic until fragrant.
4. After that, add the carrots, celery, potatoes, and peas. Stir-fry the vegetables for 2 minutes.
5. Then pour in the water and season with soy sauce, salt, and pepper. Add the tomato paste.
6. Now close the lid and set the vent to the Sealing position.
7. Press the Meat/Stew button and adjust the cooking time to 20 minutes.
8. Do quick pressure release.
9. Once the lid is open, press the Sauté button and stir in the cornstarch slurry and cook for 5 minutes until the sauce thickens.

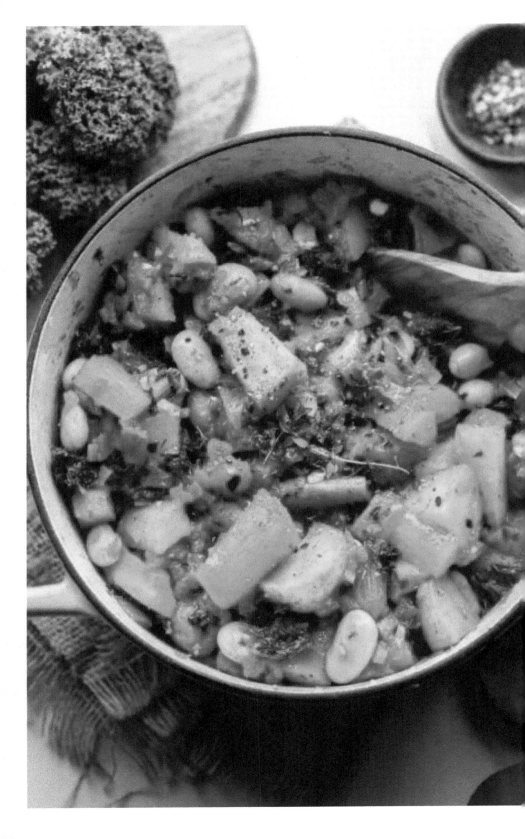

Tasty Root Vegetable and Squash Stew

Servings: 10

Preparation Time: 5 minutes

Per Serving: Calories 122, Total Fat 3g, Saturated Fat 1g, Total Carbs 24g, Net Carbs 21g, Protein 1g, Sugar: 15g, Fiber: 3g, Sodium: 53mg, Potassium: 323mg, Phosphorus: 55mg

Ingredients:

- 2 red onions
- 1 small celeriac, sliced
- 2 tablespoons tomato puree
- 2 sweet potatoes, peeled and cubed
- 4 carrots, peeled and cubed
- 2 tablespoons plain flour + 2 tablespoons cold water
- 2 teaspoons red wine vinegar
- 2 teaspoons dried thyme
- 2 tablespoons olive oil
- 2 bay leaves
- 1 butternut squash, seeded and sliced into chunks
- 2 cups plum tomatoes, chopped
- Salt and pepper to taste

Procedure:

1. First, press the Sauté button on the Instant Pot and heat the oil. Sauté the onion and celeriac. Stir for 3 minutes.
2. Now add in the squash, sweet potato, and carrots. Stir for another minute.
3. Then stir in the red wine vinegar, thyme, bay leaf, tomato puree, and tomatoes. Season with salt and pepper to taste. Add a cup of water.
4. Close the lid and set the vent to the Sealing position.
5. Now press the Meat/Stew button and adjust the cooking time to 20 minutes.
6. Do quick pressure release.
7. Once the lid is open, press the Sauté button and stir in the flour slurry.
8. In the end, cook for another 3 minutes until the sauce thickens.

Homemade Mediterranean Vegetable Stew

Servings: 8

Preparation Time: 30 minutes

Ingredients:

- 2 tbsps minced cilantro for garnish
- 2 onions, chopped
- 4 carrots, chopped
- 1 tsp ground cumin
- 2 (31-oz) can chickpeas, drained
- 1 tsp paprika
- 1 tsp saffron
- 2 (30-oz) can diced tomatoes
- 4 tbsps olive oil
- 1 head broccoli, cut into florets
- 4 cups winter squash, chopped
- 2 russet potatoes, cubed
- 3 cups vegetable broth
- 1 cup toasted slivered almonds
- 1 tsp ground ginger
- 2 tsps lemon zest
- Salt and black pepper to taste
- 1 cup pitted green olives

Procedure:

1. Take a pot and heat the oil in a pot over medium heat.

2. Then place onions and carrots and sauté for 5 minutes.
3. Now add in cumin, ginger, paprika, salt, pepper, and saffron, and cook for 30 seconds.
4. Start stirring in tomatoes, broccoli, squash, potato, chickpeas, and broth.
5. Then bring to a boil, then lower the heat and simmer for 20 minutes.
6. Now add in olives and lemon zest and simmer for 2-3 minutes.
7. Finally, garnish with cilantro and almonds to serve.

Special Chili Cannellini Bean Stew

Servings: 8

Preparation Time: 40 minutes

Ingredients:

- 2 onions, chopped
- 2 cups vegetable broth
- 4 (31-oz) cans cannellini beans
- 2 cups frozen peas, thawed
- 4 tbsps tamarind paste
- 2 (8-oz) can mild chopped green chilies
- Salt and black pepper to taste
- 1/2 cup pure agave syrup
- 2 (56-oz) can crushed tomatoes
- 4 tbsps chili powder
- 2 tsps ground coriander
- 1 tsp ground cumin
- 4 tbsps olive oil
- 4 potatoes, chopped

Procedure:

1. First, heat the oil in a pot over medium heat.
2. Then place in the onion and sauté for 3 minutes until translucent.
3. Stir in potatoes, beans, tomatoes, and chilies.
4. Now cook for 5 minutes more.

5. Take a bowl, whisk the tamarind paste with agave syrup and broth.
6. Then pour the mixture into the pot.
7. Stir in chili powder, coriander, cumin, salt, and pepper.
8. Then bring to a boil, then lower the heat and simmer for 20 minutes until the potatoes are tender.
9. Now add in peas and cook for another 5 minutes.
10. Lastly, serve warm.

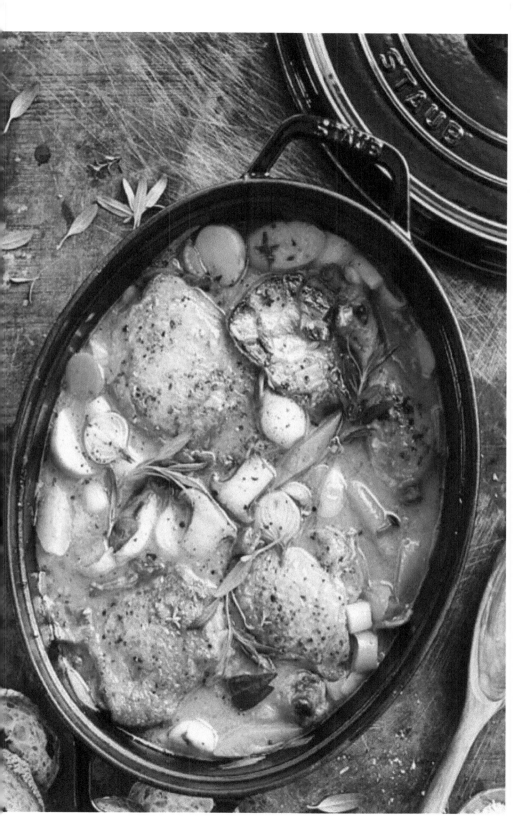

Tasty Fall Medley Stew

Servings: 8

Preparation Time: 65 minutes

Ingredients

- 2 russet potatoes, chopped
- 2 carrots, chopped
- 2 parsnips, chopped
- 2 (30-oz) can diced tomatoes
- 2 heads of savoy cabbage, chopped
- 2 cups butternut squash, cubed
- 1 cup crumbled angel hair pasta
- 1 cup dry white wine
- 4 cups vegetable broth
- 2 (31-oz) can white beans
- 1 tsp dried thyme
- 2 leeks, chopped
- 16 oz. seitan, cubed
- 4 garlic cloves, minced
- 4 tbsps olive oil

Procedure:

1. Start heating oil in a pot over medium heat.
2. Then place in seitan and cook for 3 minutes.
3. Sprinkle with salt and pepper.
4. Now add in leek and garlic and cook for another 3 minutes.

5. Aft that stirs in potato, carrot, parsnip, and squash, cook for 10 minutes.
6. Now add in cabbage, tomatoes, white beans, broth, wine, thyme, salt, and pepper.
7. Then bring to a boil, lower the heat and simmer for 15 minutes.
8. Finally, put in the pasta and cook for 5 minutes.

MAIN DISHES

Homemade Quinoa a la Putinesque

Servings: 8

Preparation Time: 30 minutes

Ingredients:

- 1/4 tsp salt
- 4 garlic cloves, minced
- 8 cups plum tomatoes, chopped
- 8 pitted green olives, sliced
- 8 pitted Kalamata olives, sliced
- 4 cups water
- 2 tbsps olive oil
- 2 tbsps chopped fresh parsley
- 3 tbsps capers, rinsed and drained
- ½ cup chopped fresh basil
- 2 cups brown quinoa
- 1/4 tsps red chili flakes

Procedure:

1. Now add quinoa, water, and salt to a medium pot and cook for 15 minutes.
2. Take a bowl, mix tomatoes, green olives, olives, capers, garlic, olive oil, parsley, basil, and red chili flakes.
3. After that, allow sitting for 5 minutes.
4. Then serve the puttanesca with the quinoa.

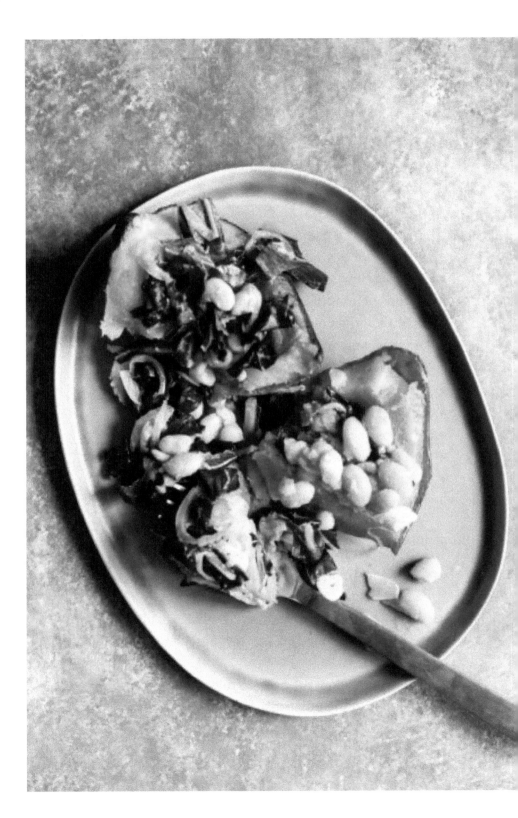

Healthy Acorn Squash Stuffed with Beans & Spinach

Servings: 8

Preparation time: 60 minutes

Ingredients:

- 2 cups chopped spinach leaves
- 4 tbsps olive oil
- 6 garlic cloves, minced
- 2 (30 oz.) can white beans, drained
- 1 cup vegetable stock
- 4 lbs. large acorn squash
- 1 tsp cumin powder
- Salt and black pepper to taste
- 1 tsp chili powder

Procedure:

1. Preheat the oven to 350 F.
2. Then cut the squash in half and scoop out the seeds. Season with salt and pepper and place face down on a sheet pan.
3. Now bake for 45 minutes.
4. Then heat olive oil in a pot over medium heat. Sauté garlic until fragrant, 30 seconds and mix in beans and spinach, allow wilting for 2 minutes, and season with salt, black pepper, cumin powder, and chili powder.

5. Now cook for 2 minutes and turn the heat off. When the squash is fork-tender, remove it from the oven and fill the holes with the bean and spinach mixture.
6. Lastly, serve.

Amazing Cabbage & Bean Stir-Fry

Servings: 4

Preparation time: 20 minutes

Ingredients:

- 1/2 cup fresh cilantro, chopped
- 2 tsps olive oil
- 4 carrots, julienned
- 2 red bell pepper, sliced
- 4 scallions, chopped
- 6 tbsp fresh mint, chopped
- 2 cups bean sprouts
- 1/2cup peanut sauce
- Fresh lime wedges
- 2 cups canned white beans
- 2 cups sliced red cabbage
- 4 tbsps roasted peanuts, chopped

Procedure:

1. Start with heating oil in a skillet and cook carrots, cabbage, and bell pepper for 10-15 minutes.
2. Stir in scallions, mint, and bean sprouts, cook for 1-2 minutes.
3. Now remove to a bowl.
4. Then mix in white beans and peanut sauce; toss to combine.
5. Garnish with cilantro and peanuts.
6. In the end, serve with lime wedges on the side.

Special Indian China Masala

Servings: 8

Preparation Time: 15 minutes

Per serving: Calories: 305; Fat: 17.1g; Carbs: 30.1g; Protein: 9.4g

Ingredients

- 2 Kashmiri chili pepper, chopped
- 2 cups tomatoes, pureed
- 2 large shallot, chopped
- 2 teaspoons fresh ginger, peeled and grated
- 8 tablespoons olive oil
- 4 cloves of garlic, minced
- 2 teaspoons coriander seeds
- Sea salt and ground black pepper, to taste
- 2 teaspoons garam masala
- 2 tablespoons fresh lime juice
- 1 teaspoon turmeric powder
- 1 cup vegetable broth
- 32 ounces canned chickpeas

Procedure:

1. Take your blender or food processor, blend the tomatoes, Kashmiri chile pepper, shallot and ginger into a paste.

2. In a saucepan, heat the olive oil over medium heat. Once hot, cook the prepared paste and garlic for about 2 minutes.
3. Now add in the remaining spices, broth and chickpeas.
4. Then turn the heat to a simmer.
5. Continue to simmer for 8 minutes more or until cooked through.
6. Now remove from the heat. Finally drizzle fresh lime juice over the top of each serving. Bon appétit!

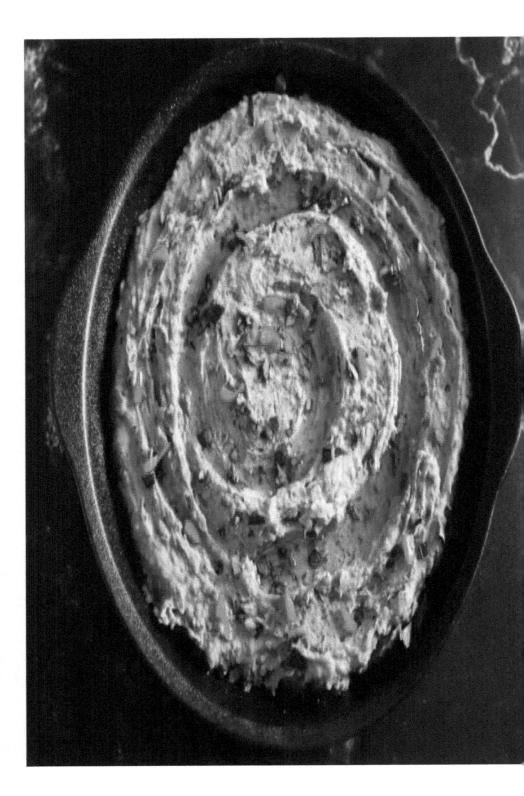

Easy Red Kidney Bean Pâté

Serving: 8

Preparation Time: 10 minutes

Per serving: Calories: 135; Fat: 12.1g; Carbs: 4.4g; Protein: 1.6g

Ingredients

- 2 onions, chopped
- 4 tablespoons olive oil
- Sea salt and ground black pepper, to taste
- 4 cloves of garlic, minced
- 2 bell peppers, chopped
- 1/2 cup olive oil
- 4 cups red kidney beans, boiled and drained
- 2 teaspoons stone-ground mustard
- 4 tablespoons fresh parsley, chopped
- 4 tablespoons fresh basil, chopped

Procedure:

1. Take a saucepan, heat the olive oil over medium-high heat.
2. Now, cook the onion, pepper and garlic until just tender or about 3 minutes.
3. Now add the sautéed mixture to your blender; now add in the remaining ingredients.
4. Then puree the ingredients in your blender or food processor until smooth and creamy.

Homemade Brown Lentil Bowl

Servings: 8

Preparation Time: 20 minutes + chilling time

Per serving: Calories: 452; Fat: 16.6g; Carbs: 61.7g; Protein: 16.4g

Ingredients

- 1 teaspoon dried oregano
- 4 cups water
- 4 cups brown rice, cooked
- 2 zucchinis, diced
- 2 red onions, chopped
- 2 teaspoons garlic, minced
- 2 cucumbers, sliced
- 2 bell peppers, sliced
- 2 cups brown lentils, soaked overnight and drained
- 8 tablespoons olive oil
- 4 cups Romaine lettuce, torn into pieces
- 2 tablespoons rice vinegar
- 4 tablespoons lemon juice
- 1 teaspoon ground cumin
- 4 tablespoons soy sauce
- Sea salt and ground black pepper, to taste
- 4 cups arugula

Procedure:

1. Now add the brown lentils and water to a saucepan and then bring to a boil over high heat.
2. Then, turn the heat to a simmer and continue to cook for 20 minutes or until tender.
3. After that place the lentils in a salad bowl and let them cool completely.
4. Now add in the remaining ingredients and toss to combine well.
5. Finally, serve at room temperature or well-chilled. Bon appétit!

Tasty Hot and Spicy Anasazi Bean Soup

Servings: 10

Preparation Time: 1 hour 10 minutes

Per serving: Calories: 352; Fat: 8.5g; Carbs: 50.1g; Protein: 19.7g

Ingredients

- 4 bell peppers, chopped
- 16 cups water
- 4 bay leaves
- 6 tablespoons olive oil
- 4 cups Anasazi beans, soaked overnight, drained and rinsed
- Sea salt and ground black pepper, to taste
- 4 medium onions, chopped
- 2 habanero peppers, chopped
- 6 cloves garlic, pressed or minced

Procedure:

1. Take a soup pot, and then bring the Anasazi beans and water to a boil.
2. Once boiling, turn the heat to a simmer.
3. Now add in the bay leaves and let it cook for about 1 hour or until tender.
4. Meanwhile, in a heavy-bottomed pot, heat the olive oil over medium-high heat. Now, sauté the

onion, peppers and garlic for about 4 minutes until tender.
5. Now add the sautéed mixture to the cooked beans.
6. Season with salt and black pepper.
7. Then continue to simmer, stirring periodically, for 10 minutes more or until everything is cooked through. Bon appétit!

Healthy n Delicious Black-Eyed Pea Salad (Ñebbe)

Servings: 10

Preparation Time: 1 hour

Per serving: Calories: 471; Fat: 17.5g; Carbs: 61.5g; Protein: 20.6g

Ingredients:

- 2 Scotch bonnet chili peppers, seeded and finely chopped
- 4 tablespoons parsley leaves, chopped
- 2 avocados, peeled, pitted and sliced
- 2 shallots, chopped
- 4 cups dried black-eyed peas, soaked overnight and drained
- 2 cucumbers, sliced
- 4 bell peppers, seeded and diced
- 4 tablespoons basil leaves,
- 2 cups cherry tomatoes, quartered
- 1/2 cup extra-virgin olive oil
- Sea salt and ground black pepper, to taste
- 4 tablespoons fresh lime juice
- 2 tablespoons apple cider vinegar

Procedure:

1. Cover the black-eyed peas with water by 2 inches and then bring to a gentle boil.
2. Let it boil for about 15 minutes.
3. Then, turn the heat to a simmer for about 45 minutes.
4. Let it cool completely.
5. Place the black-eyed peas in a salad bowl.
6. Now add in the basil, parsley, shallot, cucumber, bell peppers, cherry tomatoes, salt, and black pepper.
7. Take a mixing bowl, whisk the lime juice, vinegar, and olive oil.
8. In the end, dress the salad, garnish with fresh avocado, and serve immediately. Bon appétit!

Special Lemon Parsley Pasta

Servings: 4

Preparation Time: 10 minutes

Per Serving: Calories 377, Total Fat 17. 4g Saturated Fat 11. 9g, Cholesterol 74mg, Sodium 306mg, Total Carbohydrate 40. 7g, Dietary Fiber 1. 5g, Total Sugars 1. 2g, and Protein 17. 3g

Ingredients:

- 4 tablespoons parmesan cheese
- Enough water
- 1 cup fresh parsley, finely chopped
- 2 lemons zest
- 2 cups ziti pasta
- 3 tablespoons coconut oil
- 1 tablespoon butter
- Salt and fresh black pepper
- 2 teaspoons garlic powder

Procedure:

1. Now add butter to the Instant Pot, hit "Sauté," and once the butter is melted and sizzled.
2. Then add parsley, lemon zest, garlic powder, coconut oil, salt, and black pepper.
3. Lock the lid and make sure the vent is closed.
4. Now add water and ziti pasta.

5. Set Instant Pot to Manual or Pressure Cook on High PRESSURE for 10 minutes.
6. When cooking time ends, release pressure and wait for steam to completely stop before opening the lid.
7. After that, stir in cheese.
8. Finally, serve and enjoy.

Creamy Tofu Marsala Homemade Pasta

Servings: 4

Preparation Time: 10 minutes

Per Serving: Calories 510, Total Fat 20. 6g, Saturated Fat 14. 8g, Cholesterol 7mg, Sodium 432mg, Total Carbohydrate 45. 9g, Dietary Fiber 4. 8g, Total Sugars 7. 8g, Protein 19. 1g

Ingredients:

- 2 tablespoons coconut oil
- 1 cup grated goat cheese
- 2 small onions, diced
- 4 cups mushrooms, sliced
- 1/2 cup butter
- 1/2 cup coconut cream
- 2 cups of white wine
- 1 teaspoon garlic powder
- 3 cups of vegetable broth
- 1 cup tofu, diced into chunks
- 1 cup sun-dried tomatoes
- 2 cups fusilli

Procedure:

1. Now add the butter to the Instant Pot. Hit "Sauté."

2. Then add the onion and mushrooms and cook for 3-5 minutes, until the mushrooms have softened and browned a bit.
3. Now add the tofu and the coconut oil from the sun-dried tomatoes and cook for another 2-3 minutes until the tofu is slightly white.
4. Toss in the garlic powder and cook for 1 more minute and then add in the white wine and let it simmer for 1 minute more.
5. Now add in the vegetable broth and stir together well.
6. After that, pour in the fusilli so it's laying on top of the broth, gently smoothing and pushing it down with a spatula so it's submerged, but do not stir it with the rest of the broth.
7. Secure the lid and hit "Manual" or "Pressure Cook" High Pressure for 6 minutes. Quick-release when done and give it all a good stir.
8. Start stirring in the coconut cream and goat cheese. Let it sit for about 5 minutes, stirring occasionally, and it will thicken up into an incredible sauce, coating all the pasta perfectly.
9. Then transfer to a serving bowl, plate it up, and sprinkle any extra goat cheese if desired.

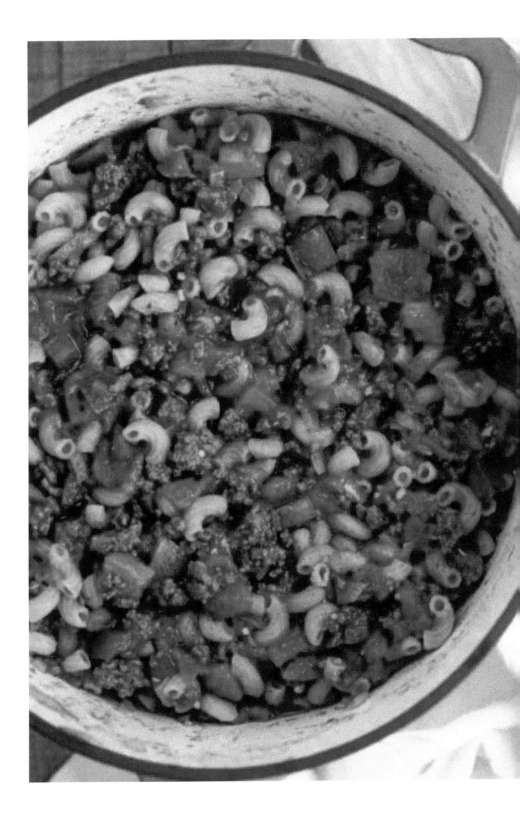

Special Classic Goulash

Servings: 4

Preparation Time: 10 minutes

Per Serving: Calories 425, Total Fat 7. 5g, Saturated Fat 1. 2g, Cholesterol 0mg, Sodium 647mg, Total Carbohydrate 73. 5g, Dietary Fiber 10. 7g, Total Sugars 24. 3g, Protein 23. 8g

Ingredients:

- 4 onions, chopped
- 3 tablespoons soy sauce
- 2 teaspoons garlic powder
- 2 cups crumbled tofu
- 2 cups uncooked elbow macaroni
- 4 cups of water
- 2 cups tomato paste
- 2 cups diced tomatoes
- 1 tablespoon dried basil
- 2 bay leaf
- 1/2 tablespoon seasoned salt, or to taste

Procedure:

1. Set Instant Pot to Sauté. Now add crumbled tofu.
2. Now add the onions and garlic powder and cook for 2 minutes. Stir regularly.

3. Start stirring the water, tomato paste, diced tomatoes, soy sauce, dried basil, bay leaf, and seasoned salt into the tofu mixture.
4. Then stir macaroni into the mixture, Secure the lid, and hit "Manual" or "Pressure Cook" High
5. Pressure for 6 minutes. Quick-release when done.

Tasty Penne with Spicy Vodka Tomato Cream Sauce

Servings: 4

Preparation Time: 10 minutes

Per Serving: Calories 394, Total Fat 28. 7g, Saturated Fat 24. 6g, Cholesterol 23mg, Sodium 720mg, Total Carbohydrate 27g, Dietary Fiber 3. 6g, Total Sugars 5. 9g, Protein 6. 8g

Ingredients:
- 1/4 cup coconut oil
- 1/4 cup chopped fresh cilantro
- 1 teaspoon garlic powder
- ½ teaspoon paprika
- 1 cup coconut cream
- 1 cup uncooked penne pasta
- 1 cup crushed tomatoes
- 2 tablespoons vodka
- Enough water
- 1 teaspoon salt

Procedure:

1. Now add penne pasta, coconut oil, water, paprika, crushed tomatoes, vodka, garlic powder, and salt to Instant Pot.
2. Then place the lid on the pot and lock it into place to seal.

3. Pressure Cook on High Pressure for 4 minutes. Use Quick Pressure Release.
4. Start stirring coconut cream into penne pasta and then stir in the fresh cilantro and combine.

Creamy Pesto Tofu

Servings: 4

Preparation Time: 10 minutes

Per Serving: Calories 711, Total Fat 62. 3g Saturated Fat 52. 7g, Cholesterol 15mg, Sodium 77mg, Total Carbohydrate 32. 5g, Dietary Fiber 6. 8g, Total Sugars 8. 8g, Protein 15. 6g

Ingredients:

- Enough water
- 1 teaspoon ground black pepper
- 1/2 cup basil pesto
- 1/2 cup grated mozzarella cheese
- 1 cup vermicelli pasta
- 1 cup tofu, peeled
- 1/2 cup butter

Procedure:

1. Set the Instant Pot to Sauté. Now add butter and wait one minute to heat up.
2. Now add the tofu, basil pesto sauté for one minute. Stir often.
3. Now add water, vermicelli pasta, and pepper.
4. Then place the lid on the pot and lock it into place to seal. Pressure Cook on High

5. Pressure for 4 minutes. Use Quick Pressure Release.
6. Put some mozzarella cheese.
7. Finally, serve and enjoy.

SWEET TREATS

Special Oatmeal Cookies with Hazelnuts

Servings: 4

Preparation Time: 15 minutes

Ingredients

- 4 tsps pure vanilla extract
- 1 cup plant butter, melted
- 1 cup pure maple syrup
- 3 cups old-fashioned oats
- 2 tsps baking powder
- 1/4 tsp salt
- 2 tsps ground cinnamon
- 1/2 tsp ground nutmeg
- 3 cups whole-grain flour
- 2 cups chopped hazelnuts
- 1/2 cup pure date sugar

Procedure:

1. Preheat oven to 360 F.
2. Then combine the flour, baking powder, salt, cinnamon, and nutmeg in a bowl.
3. Now add in oats and hazelnuts. Take another bowl; whisk the butter, maple syrup, sugar, and vanilla.
4. Then pour over the flour mixture.
5. Mix well. Spoon a small ball of cookie dough on a baking sheet and press down with a fork. Now bake for 10-12 minutes, until browned.
6. Leave it completely to cool on a rack.

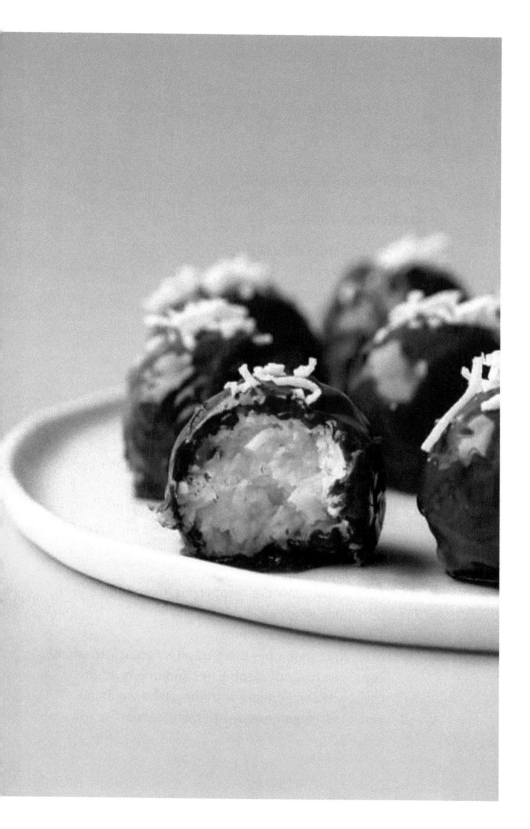

Layered Special Raspberry & Tofu Cups

Servings: 8

Preparation Time: 60 minutes

Ingredients

- 6 tbsps pure date sugar
- 1 cup soy milk
- 2 tsps vanilla extract
- 4 cups sliced raspberries
- Fresh mint leaves
- 1 cup unsalted raw cashews
- 2/4 cups firm silken tofu, drained
- 2 tsps fresh lemon juice

Procedure:

1. Grind the cashews and 3 tbsps of date sugar in a blender until a fine powder is obtained.
2. Then pour in soy milk and blitz until smooth.
3. Now add in tofu and vanilla and pulse until creamy.
4. Now remove to a bowl and refrigerate covered for 30 minutes.
5. Take a bowl; mix the raspberries, lemon juice, and remaining date sugar.
6. Then let sit for 20 minutes.
7. After that, assemble them by alternating into small cups, one layer of raspberries and one layer of cashew cream, ending with the cashew cream.
8. Finally serve garnished with mint leaves.

Delicious Cashew & Cranberry Truffles

Servings: 8

Preparation Time: 15 minutes

Ingredients

- 4 tbsps pure date sugar
- 4 tbsps pure date syrup
- 2 tsps vanilla extract
- 32 oz. cashew cream
- 4 cups fresh cranberries
- 8 tbsps plant butter
- 6 tbsps unsweetened cocoa powder

Procedure:

1. Put a silicone egg tray aside.
2. Then puree the cranberries, date syrup, and vanilla in a blender until smooth.
3. Now add the cashew cream and plant butter to a medium pot.
4. Heat over medium heat until the mixture is well combined.
5. Turn the heat off. After that, mix in the cranberry mixture and divide the mixture into the muffin holes.
6. Now refrigerate for 40 minutes or until firm.

7. Then remove the tray and pop out the truffles.
8. Meanwhile, mix the cocoa powder and date sugar on a plate.
9. In the end, roll the truffles in the mixture until well dusted and serve.

Delicious Raw Raspberry Cheesecake

Servings: 18

Preparation Time: 15 minutes chilling time

Per serving: Calories: 385; Fat: 22.9; Carbs: 41.1g; Protein: 10.8g

Ingredients:

Crust:

- 2 cups fresh dates, pitted
- 4 cups almonds
- 1/2 teaspoon ground cinnamon

Filling:

- 16 fresh dates, pitted
- 28 ounces blackberries, frozen
- 2 tablespoons fresh lime juice
- 1/2 teaspoon crystallized ginger
- 2 cans of coconut cream
- 4 cups raw cashews, soaked overnight and drained

Procedure:

1. In your food processor, blend the crust ingredients until the mixture comes together; press the crust into a lightly oiled spring-form pan.
2. Then, blend the filling layer until completely smooth.

3. Now spoon the filling onto the crust, creating a flat surface with a spatula.
4. After that, transfer the cake to your freezer for about 3 hours.
5. Store in your freezer.
6. Finally, garnish with organic citrus peel. Bon appétit!

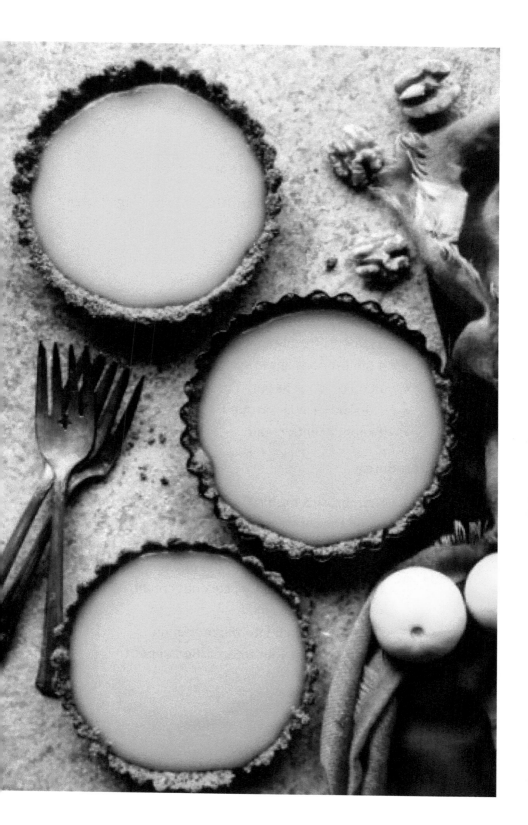

Easy Mini Lemon Tarts

Servings: 18

Preparation Time: 15 minutes+ chilling time

Per serving: Calories: 257; Fat: 16.5; Carbs: 25.4g; Protein: 4g

Ingredients:

- 2 cups dates, pitted
- 2 cups cashews
- 6 lemons, freshly squeezed
- 4 tablespoons agave syrup
- 1 cup coconut flakes
- 1 teaspoon anise, ground
- 2 cups coconut cream

Procedure:

1. First, brush a muffin tin with nonstick cooking oil.
2. Blend the cashews, dates, coconut, and anise in your food processor or a high-speed blender.
3. Now press the crust into the peppered muffin tin.
4. Then, blend the lemon, coconut cream, and agave syrup.
5. Spoon the cream into the muffin tin.
6. Lastly, store in your freezer. Bon appétit!

Healthy Fluffy Coconut Blondies with Raisins

Servings: 18

Preparation Time: 30 minutes

Per serving: Calories: 365; Fat: 18.5; Carbs: 49g; Protein: 2.1g

Ingredients

- 2 cups raisins, soaked for 15 minutes
- 2 cups all-purpose flour
- 1 teaspoon baking powder
- 2 cups coconut flour
- 1/2 teaspoon salt
- 2 cups desiccated coconut, unsweetened
- 3 cups brown sugar
- 2/4 cups vegan butter, softened
- 6 tablespoons applesauce
- 1 teaspoon vanilla extract
- 1 teaspoon ground anise

Procedure:

1. Start by preheating your oven to 350 degrees F.
2. Brush a baking pan with nonstick cooking oil.
3. Then combine the flour, baking powder, salt, and coconut.
4. Then take another bowl, mix the butter, sugar, applesauce, vanilla and anise.

5. Now stir the butter mixture into the dry ingredients; stir to combine well.
6. Fold in the raisins.
7. Then press the batter into the prepared baking pan.
8. Bake for approximately 25 minutes or until it is set in the middle.
9. At last, place the cake on a wire rack to cool slightly.

Easy Chocolate Squares

Servings: 40

Preparation Time: 1 hour 10 minutes

Per serving: Calories: 187; Fat: 13.8g; Carbs: 15.1g; Protein: 2.9g

Ingredients:

- 2 cups almond butter
- 1/2 teaspoon ground cloves
- 1/2 cup coconut oil, melted
- 1/2 cup raw cacao powder
- 1/2 teaspoon ground cinnamon
- 4 ounces dark chocolate
- 8 tablespoons agave syrup
- 2 cups cashew butter
- 2 teaspoons vanilla paste

Procedure:

1. Start with processing all the ingredients in your blender until uniform and smooth.
2. Now scrape the batter into a parchment-lined baking sheet.
3. Then place it in your freezer for at least 1 hour to set.
4. Finally, cut into squares and serve. Bon appétit!

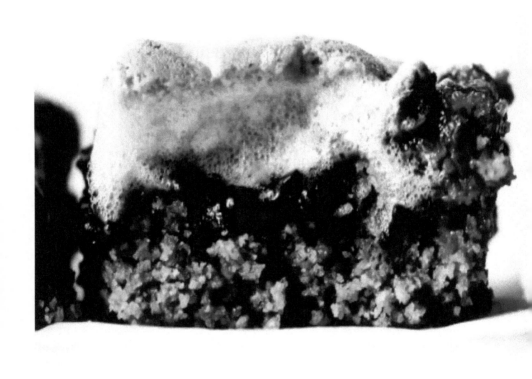

Chocolate and Raisin Tasty Cookie Bars

Servings: 20

Preparation Time: 40 minutes

Per serving: Calories: 267; Fat: 2.9g; Carbs: 61.1g; Protein: 2.2g

Ingredients;

- 4 cups almond flour
- 2 cups agave syrup
- 2 teaspoons pure vanilla extract
- 2 cups vegan chocolate, broken into chunks
- 1 cup peanut butter, at room temperature
- 1/2 teaspoon kosher salt
- 2 teaspoons baking soda
- 2 cups raisins

Procedure:

1. Take a mixing bowl; thoroughly combine the peanut butter, agave syrup, vanilla, and salt.
2. Gradually stir in the almond flour and baking soda and stir to combine.
3. Then now add in the raisins and chocolate chunks and stir again.
4. Finally, freeze for about 30 minutes and serve well chilled. Enjoy!

Delicious Raw Raspberry Cheesecake

Servings: 18

Preparation Time: 15 minutes chilling time

Per serving: Calories: 385; Fat: 22.9; Carbs: 41.1g; Protein: 10.8g

Ingredients:

Crust:

- 2 cups fresh dates, pitted
- 4 cups almonds
- 1/2 teaspoon ground cinnamon

Filling:

- 16 fresh dates, pitted
- 4 cups raw cashews, soaked overnight and drained
- 2 tablespoons fresh lime juice
- 28 ounces blackberries, frozen
- 1/2 teaspoon crystallized ginger
- 2 cans coconut cream

Procedure:

1. In your food processor, blend the crust ingredients until the mixture comes together; press the crust into a lightly oiled spring-form pan.
2. Then, blend the filling layer until completely smooth.

3. Now spoon the filling onto the crust, creating a flat surface with a spatula.
4. Transfer the cake to your freezer for about 3 hours.
5. Then store in your freezer.
6. Lastly, garnish with organic citrus peel. Bon appétit!

Healthy Fluffy Coconut Blondies with Raisins

Servings: 18

Preparation Time: 30 minutes

Per serving: Calories: 365; Fat: 18.5; Carbs: 49g; Protein: 2.1g

Ingredients

- 2 cups all-purpose flour
- 1 teaspoon baking powder
- 1/2 teaspoon salt
- 2 cups coconut flour
- 2 cups raisins, soaked for 15 minutes
- 2/4 cups vegan butter, softened
- 2 cups desiccated coconut, unsweetened
- 3 cups brown sugar
- 6 tablespoons applesauce
- 1 teaspoon vanilla extract
- 1 teaspoon ground anise

Procedure:

1. Start by preheating your oven to 350 degrees F.
2. Brush a baking pan with nonstick cooking oil.
3. Make sure to thoroughly combine the flour, baking powder, salt, and coconut. Take another bowl; mix the butter, sugar, applesauce, vanilla, and anise.

4. Then stir the butter mixture into the dry ingredients; stir to combine well.
5. Fold in the raisins.
6. Now press the batter into the prepared baking pan.
7. Bake for approximately 25 minutes or until it is set in the middle.
8. Then place the cake on a wire rack to cool slightly.

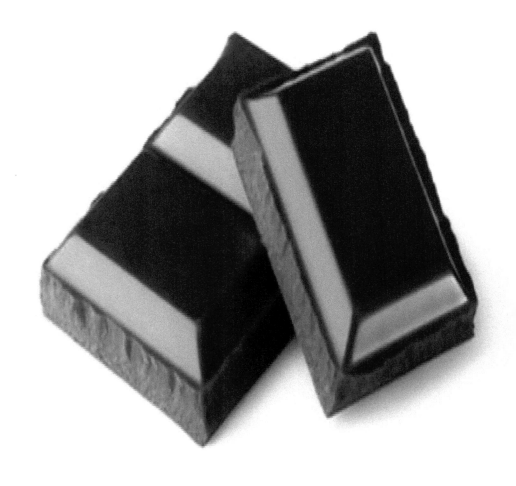

Easy Chocolate Squares

Servings: 40

Preparation Time: 1 hour 10 minutes

Per serving: Calories: 187; Fat: 13.8g; Carbs: 15.1g; Protein: 2.9g

Ingredients

- 8 tablespoons agave syrup
- 2 cups cashew butter
- 2 cups almond butter
- 1/2 teaspoon ground cloves
- 1/2 cup coconut oil, melted
- 1/2 cup raw cacao powder
- 4 ounces dark chocolate
- 2 teaspoons vanilla paste
- 1/2 teaspoon ground cinnamon

Procedure:

1. Start with processing all the ingredients in your blender until uniform and smooth.
2. Then scrape the batter into a parchment-lined baking sheet.
3. Now place it in your freezer for at least 1 hour to set.
4. Lastly, cut into squares and serve. Bon appétit!

Homemade Chocolate and Raisin Cookie Bars

Servings: 20

Preparation Time: 40 minutes

Per serving: Calories: 267; Fat: 2.9g; Carbs: 61.1g; Protein: 2.2g

Ingredients:

- 2 cups raisins
- 2 cups agave syrup
- 2 cups vegan chocolate, broken into chunks
- 2 teaspoons pure vanilla extract
- 1 cup peanut butter, at room temperature
- 1/2 teaspoon kosher salt
- 4 cups almond flour
- 2 teaspoons baking soda

Procedure:

1. Take a mixing bowl; thoroughly combine the peanut butter, agave syrup, vanilla, and salt.
2. Gradually stir in the almond flour and baking soda and stir to combine.
3. After that, now add in the raisins and chocolate chunks and stir again.
4. Then freeze for about 30 minutes and serve well chilled. Enjoy!

Delicious Chocolate Mousse Cake

Servings: 8

Preparation Time: 15-30 minutes

Per Serving: Calories 608 Fats 60. 5g Carbs 19. 8g Protein 6.3g

Ingredients:

- 1/2 cup unsalted plant butter, melted
- Fresh raspberries or strawberries for topping
- 1 1/3 cups toasted almond flour
- 4 cups unsweetened chocolate bars, broken into pieces
- 5 cups coconut cream

Procedure:

1. Start with lightly greasing a 9-inch spring-form pan with some plant butter and set aside.
2. Mix the almond flour and plant butter in a medium bowl and pour the mixture into the spring-form pan.
3. Then use the spoon to spread and press the mixture into the bottom of the pan.
4. Now place in the refrigerator to firm for 30 minutes.

5. Meanwhile, pour the chocolate into a safe microwave bowl and melt for 1 minute stirring every 30 seconds.
6. After that, remove from the microwave and mix in the coconut cream and maple syrup.
7. Also, remove the cake pan from the oven, pour the chocolate mixture on top, making sure to shake the pan and even the layer.
8. Chill further for 4 to 6 hours.
9. Take out the pan from the fridge, release the cake and garnish with the raspberries or strawberries.
10. In the end, slice and serve.

Homemade Apple Raspberry Cobbler

Servings: 4

Preparation Time: 15-30 minutes

Per Serving: Calories 539 Fats 12g Carbs 105. 7g Protein 8. 2g

Ingredients:

- 4 tbsps pure date sugar
- 4 tbsps pure date sugar
- 2 tsps cinnamon powder
- 2 cups fresh raspberries
- 4 tbsps unsalted plant butter
- 6 apples, peeled, cored, and chopped
- 1 cup whole-wheat flour
- 2 cups toasted rolled oats

Procedure:

1. Preheat the oven to 350 F and grease a baking dish with some plant butter.
2. Then now add the apples, date sugar, and 3 tbsps of water to a medium pot.
3. Then cook over low heat until the date sugar melts, and then mix in the raspberries.
4. Now cook until the fruits soften, 10 minutes.
5. Pour and spread the fruit mixture into the baking dish and set aside.

6. After that, take a blender, now add the plant butter, flour, oats, date sugar, and cinnamon powder.
7. Pulse a few times until crumbly.
8. Then spoon and spread the mixture on the fruit mix until evenly layered.
9. Bake in the oven for 25 to 30 minutes or until golden brown on top.
10. Finally, remove the dessert, allow cooling for 2 minutes, and serve.

Tasty Cardamom Coconut Fat Bombs

Servings: 6

Preparation Time: 5 minutes

Per Serving: Calories: 687, Total Fat: 54.5g, Saturated Fat: 27.4 g, Total Carbs: 9g, Dietary Fiber: 2g, Sugar: 4g, Protein: 38g, Sodium: 883 mg

Ingredients:

- 6 oz. unsalted butter, room temperature
- 1/2 tsp green cardamom powder
- 1/2 tsp cinnamon powder
- 1 cup unsweetened grated coconut
- 1 tsp vanilla extract

Procedure:

1. Start with pouring the grated coconut into a skillet and roast until lightly brown. Set aside to cool.
2. Take a bowl; combine the butter, half of the coconut, cardamom, vanilla, and cinnamon.
3. Then use your hands to form bite-size balls from the mixture and roll each in the remaining coconut.
4. Now refrigerate the balls until ready to serve.

Lightning Source UK Ltd.
Milton Keynes UK
UKHW020641090421
381706UK00001B/53